CHAPTER ONE

INTRODUCTION

You tend to hear "I'm SO stressed out!" from almost everyone you know regularly. Pressures are everywhere in today's environment. These pressures lead to stress and worry, and we are frequently ill-prepared to handle the stressors that result in anxiety and other unpleasant emotions that may lead to illness. I'll, literally.

The numbers are astounding. An anxiety condition affects one in eight Americans between the ages of 18 and 54. Over 19 million people in all! Anxiety disorders are the second most common mental health issue among American women, after alcohol and drug abuse, according to research from the National Institute of Mental Health.

Compared to men, women experience worry and stress almost twice as frequently. In terms of prevalence, anxiety disorders outnumber depression as the most prevalent mental illness in America. The most prevalent mental health condition affecting persons over 65 is anxiety. Each year, anxiety problems cost the United States $46.6 billion. Patients with anxiety typically see five doctors before receiving a correct diagnosis.

Unfortunately, anxiety and stress often coexist. In actuality, anxiety is one of the main signs of stress. Additionally, stress is directly or indirectly responsible for 80 percent of all illnesses.

Stress is more harmful than we previously realized. Although you've surely heard that stress can raise blood pressure, raising the risk of a stroke in the distant future, a recent health insurance pamphlet indicated that stress-related problems accounted for 90% of visits to a primary care physician.

According to Health Psychology magazine, ongoing stress might hinder the immune system's ability to operate normally. Additionally, research has shown that people who are under stress are more prone to being sick and are also more likely to develop allergies, autoimmune, or cardiovascular disorders.

According to medical professionals, the digestive and immunological systems, as well as other bodily processes not necessary for survival, shut down under prolonged stress. People get sick because of this, he claims. Psychosomatic illness, a disease with an emotional or psychological component, is also very common.

Additionally, stress frequently causes people to react in harmful ways, such as smoking, drinking alcohol, eating badly, or engaging in inactive lifestyles. In addition to the wear and tear caused by the stress itself, this harms the body.

Stress is a natural aspect of life. Maintaining our health and well-being depends entirely on how we respond to it. Life is full of pressures, and those tensions lead to stress. You must accept that stress will always be a part of your life, but you may develop coping mechanisms to transform it into a more positive experience.

I remember thinking when I originally had the task of writing this book, "Sure, you can get rid of tension and anxiety by isolating yourself in a room and never talking to anyone again." But a book like that wouldn't be very educational, would it?

Stress-related anxiety disorders have plagued me for a long time. Despite constantly learning new topics and coping techniques, I feel like I have learned how to deal with that in some ways. To give you tools that will aid you in difficult situations, I've blended some of my own experiences with guidance from professionals in this book.

I've also provided several strategies for dealing with the crippling anxiety and panic episodes that many individuals experience. I've discovered some incredible stuff while doing research for this book, and I can't wait to share it with you. Let's look at how to get rid of tension and worry in your life because I've learned so much myself!

HOW TO GET RID OF ANXIETY AND STRESS
IN YOUR LIFE FOREVER!

THE MOST EFFECTIVE METHOD FOR
HANDLING ANXIETY, PANIC ATTACKS,
INTERNAL TERROR, AND FINDING PEACE IN A
BEAUTIFUL WORLD, THE ONLY THING THAT
MATTERS IS MANAGING YOUR EMOTIONS AT
ALL TIMES.

By George .S. Alan

I have made every reasonable effort to be as accurate and complete as possible in the creation of this book and to ensure that the information provided is free from errors; however, the author/publisher assumes no responsibility for errors, omissions, or contrary interpretation of the subject matter herein and does not warrant or represent at any time that the contents within are accurate due to the rapidly changing nature of the internet.

Contents

CHAPTER TWO

WHY ARE WE UNDER SUCH STRESS?

We are in extremely stressful and challenging times, and nothing appears to be getting any better. Even though life can often feel incredibly difficult and unfair, we manage to push through, day after day, hoping and praying that things will get better soon.

But the world is getting weirder, more unpredictable, and more stressful daily. These days, nothing feels secure. There are record numbers of people who are in debt. Many people are losing their jobs, homes, health, and occasionally even their sanity. There are far too many people who seem to live with worry, sadness, and anxiety.

The Age of Anxiety appears to have arrived. Time magazine loudly and clearly announced this as the featured subject in that issue on one of its covers in 2002. Many of us appear to lead lives marked by perpetual anxiety and concern as a result of the strain and uncertainty that come with living in the twenty-first century.

This ongoing anxiety and stress seemed to get worse after the September 11 terrorist strikes. Many individuals say they are still terrified that something of that size could occur again, possibly closer to them, four years later.

We are constantly exposed to upsetting visuals and tales when we turn on the news or open a newspaper. We start to doubt where we are safe. Never before have we had such easy access to so much information as we do in this era of information.

The economy is another source of stress. Both our nation and many Americans are in debt. Many Americans now work in monotonous and unsatisfactory occupations as a result of rising gas prices, exorbitant housing costs, and even the cost of food. They work on these tasks to support themselves. Today, it's more crucial to bring home the bacon rather than work in a dream career.

Stress is increased when there are more women in the workforce. So many women believe they must be the breadwinner, the housekeeper, the mother, the wife, the daughter, and the sister. The only issue with that is that some women simply don't carve out time for themselves, which contributes to their chronic stress.

Even young children might experience stress and worry. Teenagers who desire to attend colleges sometimes push themselves academically to attempt and get scholarships so they can attend institutions with rising tuition costs.

In addition to all of that, they find themselves needing to work part-time jobs to pay for things that their parents can no longer afford. Peer pressure makes the situation into a true pressure cooker!

With the help of cell phones, the internet, palm pilots, blackberries, and iPods, we are constantly on the move and approachable. We no longer set aside time to unwind and relish life. why not Of course we should!

We feel under pressure to carry out these actions because we believe we MUST rather than because we WANT to. People find it difficult to just say "No" far too frequently. By not speaking just one simple word, we accumulate unnecessary duties and expectations, which causes us anxiety.

Every one of us will come across circumstances that could lead to worry or anxiety. The causes are too numerous to list, but some of them include purchasing a home, having overnight guests (in-laws!), being bullied, attending exams, caring for children, handling finances, having marital problems, traveling, etc.

It's "natural" to experience stress in daily life. It doesn't become a problem until it seems to rule our life.

Everyone will feel pressure for different reasons depending on the circumstances. Generally speaking, we become anxious or tense when we don't feel in control of a situation and we can feel its grip tightening around us.

The solution is to try to change this and regain control if stress is brought on by our lack of feeling in control of a situation. You can, which is wonderful news!

You already possess all of the resources required to beat stress and the resulting worry. The issue is that because we sometimes feel so out of control, we frequently fail to recognize that we are in charge. But you only need to use the available tools.

Let's first examine the obstacles we erect that prohibit us from achieving health and overcoming our anxiety and tension.

CHAPTER THREE

BLOCKING ACTIONS MAINTAINS YOUR STRESS

You are most certainly indulging in three compulsive activities that impeded your recovery and prevent you from living a stress-free life. The first step in overcoming the issues associated with being overly stressed can be to recognize these obstacles.

Negativity obsession is the first. If you tend to be "negative" about people, places, situations, and other aspects of your life, you are said to be compulsively negative.

Sayings like "I can't do this!" or "No one understands!" or "Nothing ever works!" can come to mind. Your "sour grapes" attitude prevents you from knowing what it's like to view life from a positive perspective and appreciate the beauty in yourself and those around you, even though you could be doing it unintentionally. There is a vast universe filled with enjoyment and optimistic thoughts for you.

The next is compulsive perfectionism. Obsessive perfectionism is attempting to do everything "just so," even if it means putting yourself in a state of anxiety in the process. The ability to enjoy things without feeling "uptight" or "stressed" is severely hampered by statements such, as "I have to do this correctly, or I'll be a failure!" or "If I'm not precise, people will be upset at me!" Again, this behavior may be completely beneath the threshold of your awareness.

OCD is the last type of analysis. You find yourself wanting to revisit a task or an issue repeatedly when you are obsessed with analysis. For instance, you could catch yourself saying things like, "If I relax and let things go without giving them much thought, things go wrong!" or "I need to read this over, study it, and know it inside and out...otherwise, I can't relax!"

The ability to think analytically is a great quality, but if it dominates your life, you won't have time to stop and smell the roses because you'll be too busy trying to make sense of everything and everyone around you. One of the most crucial steps to letting go of tension and taking full control of your anxiety is gaining an understanding of this kind of conduct.

There are two things you may do to aid yourself if you catch yourself engaging in any of the aforementioned "Blocking Behaviors." Start by asking the individuals you know, love, and trust if they find you to be negative, whiny, or difficult to be around.

You might find it difficult to hear what I'm saying since the truth can often be very painful. However, the perspective you will gain from how people perceive you will be priceless, and you will be fully aware of their perceptions. Accept their advice as useful information, and be confident that you will learn a lot from what they say.

Even if you don't like the notion of writing, you can jot down brief entries each day in a notebook or diary to track trends of when you engage in "blocking behaviors" and to keep track of your progress. The best thing is that you'll start to recognize patterns in your behavior that show you exactly how you're putting off treating your anxiety.

But before you can move on to the "healing" step and overcome your stress and anxiety, you must first identify these blocks. We'll provide you with some terrific stress-busting tactics later in the book.

Many individuals believe that stress and anxiety are interchangeable terms. The opposite is true, as you can see!

CHAPTER FOUR

STRESS OR ANXIETY

Contrary to popular assumption, stress and anxiety are not synonymous. The pressures we experience in life lead to stress, which is caused by the hormone adrenaline being released. An extended period of the hormone's presence can lead to depression, an increase in blood pressure, and other undesirable changes and outcomes.

Anxiety is one of these adverse consequences. When a person has anxiety, fear takes the place of all other emotions, including concern and apprehension, leaving them isolated and jittery. Chest aches, lightheadedness, shortness of breath, and panic episodes are further symptoms.

An existing stressor or stressors are what causes stress. Stress that persists after the stressor has passed is anxiety. Any circumstance or thinking that makes you feel irritated, furious, worried, or even anxious might cause stress. Not everything that stresses out one person will necessarily stress out another.

Anxiety is a state of trepidation or worry that nearly often comes with a sense of impending disaster. The fact that you may not always be aware of the cause of your discomfort can make you feel worse.

Stress is the way that our bodies and thoughts respond to something that breaks the equilibrium of our daily lives; an example of stress is the reaction that we experience when we feel threatened or scared. The hormone adrenaline, which activates our body's defense mechanisms and causes our hearts to race, blood pressure to increase, muscles to tense, and eye pupils to widen, is released by our adrenal glands during stressful situations.

Your pulse rate increasing is one of the main signs of increased stress, but having a normal pulse doesn't mean you're not anxious. You may notice symptoms of stress such as persistent aches and pains, palpitations, worry, chronic exhaustion, sobbing, overeating or undereating, recurrent infections, and a decline in your sexual desire.

Naturally, we do not always respond in such severe ways to stress, and we are not always under as much pressure or dread when we are faced with a difficult circumstance.

Stress affects some people more than others; for some, even routine daily decisions seem impossible. For them, choosing what to eat for supper or what to buy at the supermarket presents a seemingly insurmountable challenge. On the other hand, some people appear to flourish under strain by becoming extremely productive while being propelled by pressure.

According to research, women who have children have greater blood levels of stress-related hormones than women who do not. Does this imply that women without children don't go through stressful times? Without a doubt!

It implies that women who are childless may not suffer stress as frequently or to the same degree as women who are parents. This means that scheduling time for yourself is especially crucial for women who are raising children because once your stress level is lower, you will be better able to support your kids and handle the daily challenges of being a parent.

On the other side, anxiety is a sense of unease. Everybody feels it when they are in a stressful circumstance, as right before an exam or an interview, or when they are experiencing a health concern. When facing something challenging or risky, it's acceptable to feel apprehensive, and mild anxiety might even be a good thing.

But for many people, anxiety makes daily life difficult. Excessive anxiety frequently coexists with psychiatric disorders like depression. When anxiety is exceedingly intense or persistent, occurs in the absence of a stressful incident, or interferes with regular tasks like going to work, it is deemed abnormal.

The brain sends signals to various body parts to get them ready for the "fight or flight" reaction, which results in the physical symptoms of anxiety. The body's organs that function faster include the heart, lungs, and others Adrenaline and other stress hormones are also released by the brain. The following are typical signs of excessive anxiety:

1• Diarrhea
2• Mouth dry
3• Palpitations or a rapid heartbeat
4• Insomnia
5• Intolerance or rage
6• Lack of concentration
7• The worry of going "crazy"
8• Depersonalization is the sensation of being unreal and without control over your actions.

There are numerous techniques to induce anxiety. Stress in your life can cause you to have uneasy thoughts. Many persons with anxiety problems spend a lot of time worrying excessively. This can be worrying over anything, including your health, your career, or global issues.

Certain substances, both illegal and legal, can cause withdrawal symptoms or side effects that can resemble anxiety symptoms. Caffeine, alcohol, nicotine, cold treatments, decongestants, bronchodilators for asthma, tricyclic antidepressants, cocaine, amphetamines, diet pills, ADHD meds, and thyroid medications are some examples of these substances.

Stress or anxiety can also be brought on by an unhealthy diet, such as one with insufficient vitamin B12 levels. Performance anxiety is linked to certain circumstances, such as taking a test or giving a public presentation. A stressful incident like war, physical or sexual abuse, or a natural disaster can cause post-traumatic stress disorder (PTSD), a stress disorder.

An adrenal gland tumor known as a pheochromocytoma may occasionally be the root of anxiety. The hormones that trigger anxiety-related thoughts, feelings, and behaviors are overproduced as a result of this.

Although nervousness can be a little frightening, what's much scarier is how much stress and worry can contribute to depression. I am well aware that dealing with depression can be a lifelong struggle, but the good news is that everything can be controlled!

So let's take a few quick tests to determine whether you have an excessive amount of stress, anxiety, or sadness.

QUIZ TIME!

Please be aware that we are not medical specialists before you continue. This material has been verified but is in no way intended to be a comprehensive diagnostic tool. These tests are merely guides to assist you in identifying any issues you may have and being able to successfully address those issues.

Let's start with determining whether you might be depressed because it can be the most serious of our themes. Remember that everyone experiences "blue" days occasionally. The fact that the symptoms develop gradually distinguishes clinical depression from mere melancholy. They are persistent and have the potential to negatively impact your life; they don't come and go.

Consider the following queries. If you have had these feelings consistently during the past two weeks, select yes.

1. Do you frequently feel depressed?
2. Are you lacking the motivation to perform routine tasks like taking a shower, cleaning the house, or preparing dinner?
3. Do others frequently comment on your irritability?
4. Do you find it difficult to focus?
5. Even when loved ones and friends are there, do you feel lonely?
6. Have you grown bored with your favorite pastimes?
7. Do you experience feelings of hopelessness, unworthiness, or unjustified guilt?

8. Do you struggle to fall asleep and are perpetually tired?
9. Has your weight significantly changed?

If "Yes" is your response to five or more of these inquiries, you may be experiencing clinical depression. You should look for medical assistance from a specialist, such as a doctor or a therapist. There are numerous drugs available that can treat depression.

When I started taking an anti-depressant, I tried to hide my depression but I couldn't believe what a difference just one tablet a day made! If you believe you are sad, take action right away. It helped me escape the "dark hole" I had become trapped in and helped me appreciate life again. You should be content.

Let's check to see if you're unduly stressed out, though, as this book is about stress and anxiety. Consider the following:

1. Do you frequently worry and engage in critical self-talk?
2. Do you find it difficult to focus?
3. Do you respond and get angry quickly?
4. Do you frequently have neck or head pain?
5. Are you a tooth grinder?
6. Do you experience overwhelming, anxiety, or depression frequently?
7. Do you use unhealthy coping mechanisms to deal with stress, such as bingeing on food or alcohol, smoking, arguing, or finding other methods to ignore people and life?
8. Do you find it difficult to enjoy simple pleasures?
9. Do you occasionally lose your temper over petty issues?

You have excessive stress in your life if you can "Yes" to the majority of these questions. The good news is that by purchasing this book, you will gain access to a wealth of useful stress-reduction strategies. However, we'll discuss that later.

Now let's talk about anxiety.

1. Do you ever feel out of breath, have heart palpitations, or shake while you're at rest?

2. Do you worry about losing your mind or going crazy?
3. Do you shy away from social situations out of fear?
4. Do you have any object phobias?
5. Do you worry that you'll be stuck somewhere or in a predicament that's impossible to get out of?
6. Are you terrified to leave your house?
7. Do you occasionally have persistent thoughts or visions?
8. Do you find yourself doing the same things over and over again?
9. Do you frequently think back on a distressing former experience?

More than four "Yes" responses to these questions may suggest an anxiety problem.

Your general health may be jeopardized if you experience depression, high levels of stress, or excessive worry, thus you must take action right away to overcome these issues.

Numerous physical and psychological aspects of our bodies are impacted by stress and worry. Because stress and worry induce changes in our bodies' chemical makeup, they are linked to cancer and other dangerous diseases.

Stress and anxiety don't have to control your life; all it takes is discipline and a structured plan. It would be quite helpful to avoid consuming anything that you cannot tolerate. Recognize your restrictions and abide by them. Never overwork yourself. Simply attempt to cross the border a single inch at a time.

Without putting your health at risk, you can live a successful, satisfying life and job. If not, you are not only killing yourself but also your loved ones, friends, and everyone else in your vicinity.

Life is certain to be stressful at times. It can be both physical and mental, and a lot of the time, pressures from daily life can cause it. There are differences in how each person manages stress.

However, if stress is not managed, it can lead to behavioral, mental, and physical issues that can harm your relationships at work and in your personal life as well as your health.

As previously stated, panic attacks can result from stress and anxiety. Having a panic attack can be a serious issue, as I can attest from personal experience. Let's delve a little more into that topic.

CHAPTER FIVE

PANIC ATTACKS

The terrible result of experiencing extreme stress and anxiety is that your body will respond to the situation physically. It appears as though your body is urging you to take a short break. It's anything but restful while you're experiencing a panic attack, though.

While my husband and I were returning from a St. Louis Rams football game, I experienced my first panic attack. I started to feel a little "weird" when we were approximately 30 miles from our house. My heart seemed to be beating at a speed of 90 miles per hour, I was having problems breathing, and I felt separated from my body.

I parked the van by the side of the road and got out in the hope that I might "walk it off." It didn't, though. No matter what I did, I was unable to get a breath. I thought I was going to die. I can still hear myself pleading, "Please not now. It was terrifying, and I wasn't ready.

The good news is that I certainly wasn't going to die! But that evening marked the start of a horrific exploration of how my body responded to high levels of stress and worry. Since then, I've experienced a lot of panic attacks, but I've also developed the ability to spot and manage them when they do. It's a lot better than it was, even if I can't always fully control it and occasionally have full-blown panic.

Let's now examine the warning signals of a potential panic attack. The list that follows identifies warning signals of impending panic attacks.

1• Palpitations
2• An increased heart rate or a racing heart
3• Sweating
4• Shaking or trembling
5• Breathlessness
6• A feeling of choking
7• Aches and pains in the chest
8• Vomiting or stomach pain

9• Desensitization (a feeling of unreality)
10• Apprehension of becoming crazy or losing control
11• Concern with death
12• Feeling numb or tingly in your face and limbs
13• Cold sweats or hot flashes

You'd be shocked at how often patients arrive at the emergency room of the hospital certain that they are experiencing a heart attack only to learn that it is a panic attack. They are that serious!

When you experience a panic attack, it can be very difficult for your loved ones to comprehend or even picture what you are going through. They can become impatient with you, tell you to "get over it," or suspect you of being a fake. If you show them the following situation, it might be helpful.

At the grocery store, there is a line. Even though you've been waiting for a while, there is only one more customer before you reach the cashier. What the heck was that?

Your chest tightens, an awful sensation develops in your throat, you start to feel suddenly short of breath, and, what do you know, your heart begins to miss a beat. "God, please don't be here."

You quickly survey the area to see if it poses a threat. There are four hostile faces behind you and one in front of you. You feel as though pins and needles are stabbing you through your left arm, you start to feel a little lightheaded, and then fear explodes as you prepare for the worst. A panic attack is about to happen to you.

You are now certain that this will be a significant event. Now you need to pay attention. You are aware of how to handle this, or at least you think you are! Start inhaling deeply while exhaling through your mouth.

Breathe in, repeat the word "Relax," while thinking of soothing ideas, and then exhale. However, it doesn't seem to be helping; in fact, focusing just on breathing makes you feel self-conscious and tenser.

Perhaps if you simply attempt to relax your muscles. Hold the tension in both shoulders for 10 seconds, then let go. Try it one more. Nope, there hasn't changed. The anxiety is getting worse, and the lack of effective coping mechanisms makes your terror much worse. If only your family or a close friend were there to support you, you could feel more at ease handling this circumstance.

Your body is now buzzing with unpleasant sensations, the adrenaline in your system is rushing, and you are experiencing the dreadful feeling of losing control of your emotions. Nobody nearby has any clue of the extreme terror you are going through. They view it as just another ordinary day and another interminably long grocery line.

You understand you have no other choices. Time to leave now. As it is now your moment to pay, you remove yourself from the line while still looking ashamed. As you leave your purchases behind and make your way to the door, the cashier is staring at you perplexed.

You need some alone time; there is no time for justifications. You exit the store and get in your car to drive home by yourself. You ponder whether this was the major incident. The person you fear will make you physically and mentally exhausted. The panic eases ten minutes later. How on earth are you going to get through the remainder of your day when it's just 11:00 in the morning?

The above situation undoubtedly sounds quite familiar if you frequently experience panic or anxiety attacks. Even simply reading it might have caused anxiety and fear. Even writing was challenging for me.

You could experience panic and anxiety in different situations. The physical sensations might be a little different. It's crucial to understand that panic attacks are really real to the people experiencing them, and they shouldn't ever be ignored.

One evening at home, I was alone and I was watching one of my favorite shows on television. I believed I was in a secure location. I felt fully at ease and there was no clear trigger. I suddenly started to experience the signs of a panic attack. My living room's four walls were surrounding me and enclosed me. I felt like I was going to die because I couldn't breathe.

I went outside into my front porch for some fresh air and started practicing deep breathing. Once the symptoms subsided, I began to question why exactly I had that episode. There was no evident cause, no demanding circumstance, and no sign that a panic attack might be about to occur.

The odd thing about panic is that. Your mind can trick you occasionally. Even when you believe there is little chance you may experience a panic attack, your brain may be sensing otherwise. The worrying part is that. The good news is that there are strategies to prevent panic attacks and manage them considerably better when they occur.

CHAPTER SIX

CONTROLLING PANIC ATTACKS

Knowing that you are not the only one who suffers from panic attacks may provide you some consolation. Not even one in a million people are you. Nearly 5% of the population in America is thought to have an anxiety disorder of some kind.

Some people may experience only intermittent panic attacks, such as when required to speak in front of others, while others may experience frequent, recurrent panic episodes that prevent them from leaving their homes. Frequently occurring panic attacks frequently result in what doctors refer to as an "anxiety disorder.

Managing an anxiety problem can be done in a variety of ways. Others might work for you even though some might not. Knowing some of the most popular coping mechanisms might help you deal with panic attacks as soon as they hit.

Knowing when a panic attack is about to start is the first step. Once you've had enough of them, you begin to pay close attention to the tingling sensation, the feeling of being out of breath, and the sense of being disconnected from the world around you.

Many folks I speak with are curious about that disconnect. They find it challenging to comprehend. We panic attack sufferers are all too familiar with it. It's similar to being able to perceive a solid item from a distance. Even if you are aware of its presence, you have some reservations about its veracity.

You may want to touch that thing just to make sure. You feel cut off from the environment around you. It seems as though you have no influence over anything around you and are merely a spectator in your own life.

This is a terrible feeling, I assure you.

So how do you start trying to combat your panic attacks? Would you believe me if I said that the key to stopping panic and anxiety attacks is to WANT one? Doesn't that sound odd, perhaps even contradictory? But the desire aids in driving it away.

Does this imply that you ought to be allowed to start having a panic attack right now? Without a doubt! It suggests that whatever you are scared of—in this case, a panic attack—will probably manifest and cause chaos. Your odds of repelling the attack increase when you resist it.

When you fight against anything out of fear, that fear will stay with you. How do you quit resisting? You confront the anxiety head-on, which prevents it from continuing.

In essence, this means that you cannot experience a panic attack if you intentionally seek one out every day. You cannot have a panic attack right now, I can assure you of that. You may not be aware of it, but you've always chosen to worry. Whether you say this is beyond my power consciously or unconsciously, it is your decision.

Another approach to understanding this is to compare experiencing a panic attack to being perched precariously on a precipice. You feel as though the anxiety is bringing you ever closer to losing control. You have to metaphorically jump to get over your fear. You must plunge off the cliff and into all of your greatest fears, including anxiety and fear.

Jumping technique Jumping makes you desire to experience a panic episode. You actively invite anxiety and panic episodes by going about your daily activities.

Your true sense of security comes from knowing that a panic attack can never hurt you. A medical fact is that. Although the feelings are intense, you are protected and nothing bad will happen to you. Although your heart is beating, nothing bad will happen to you. The jump reduces to a two-foot drop only! It's completely secure.

Your life becomes unbalanced as a result of anxiety because of how much mental concern you experience as a top-heavy feeling. Your entire body's center of attention is shifted to your head. Schools of meditation frequently use the ease with which the body can lose its feeling of the center as an illustration of this top-heavy imbalance.

Relaxation is the key to conquering panic attacks. It's simple to say but challenging to achieve. Focusing on your breathing and making sure it is slow and steady is a fantastic method to achieve this. Breathing problems are one of the earliest indications of a panic attack, and you can feel yourself gasping to take a breath. Your heart rate will slow and the terror will pass if you concentrate on even breathing.

A relaxing impact of slower, deeper breathing is felt. Letting all of the air out of your lungs will help you breathe more easily. This makes it difficult for your lungs to take a deep breath afterward. You'll notice that your breathing is deeper and that you feel calmer if you keep your attention on your out-breath and allow all the air out of your lungs.

The goal is to divert attention from the fact that you are experiencing a panic attack. One at a time, make an effort to drive your feet into the earth. Feel how firmly anchored to the earth they are.

Lying down with your bottom close to a wall is an even better position. Knees bowed, place your feet against the wall, and press each foot against the surface one at a time. It will work better if you can breathe in as you press your foot up against the wall and out as you let go. You ought to switch between your feet. To stop the panic, continue doing this for 10 to 15 minutes.

Consider what you see, hear, feel, and smell in your surroundings by using all of your senses. You'll be able to stay present if you do this. Typically, feelings of panic are connected to unpleasant memories of the past or unpleasant anticipations of the future. Anything that keeps your attention on the here and now will be soothing. Try petting a pet, scanning your room for colors, textures, and shapes, paying close attention to the sounds you hear, making a friend call, or simply taking in the smells around you.

Aromatherapy is enthusiastically endorsed by many people as a treatment for panic and anxiety. When you smell lavender, it can be extremely calming and soothing. Lavender essential oil is widely available in retail outlets. Keep it nearby and inhale when you begin to feel worried.

Try rubbing some oil (olive or grape seed oil will work) with a few drops of lavender essential oil in it. When not in use, keep a prepared mixture in a dark glass bottle. Even better, prepare many bottles, one of which can be tiny enough to carry anywhere.

Helichrysum, frankincense, and marjoram are further essential oils that have been shown to relieve anxiety and panic episodes. Use the oil that most appeals to you after giving each one a sniff, or a combination of your favorite oils blended with olive or grape seed oil.

You might want to get ready before having a panic attack. Make a list of the things you're worried will happen when you're not in a panic. Then jot down some calming statements that tell you to be afraid of nothing. When terror begins to set in, you might then tell yourself these things.

When you need it, you can refer to your prepared list of things to do in the event of panic. Fill it with several relaxing sayings and suggestions for calming activities. I find this to be a very useful tool, and I never leave home without my little notepad with these encouraging statements in it.

Being in a state of panic can be extremely frightening, especially if you're alone. Making plans for when the panic hits can significantly lessen and occasionally even prevent the panic.

Utilizing visualization is a fantastic additional strategy for reducing stress and anxiety.

CHAPTER SEVEN

CALM YOURSELF WITH VISUALIZATION

By using visualization, you can easily release mental tension, stress, and worrisome thoughts. When you're under pressure, you can employ visualization, and it's especially helpful when your mind is racing with scary, worried thoughts.

When used frequently, this visualization technique is particularly efficient at getting rid of persistent mental concerns or bothersome ideas. The exercise must be performed for longer than 10 minutes at a time to reap its full benefits; anything less will not produce discernible effects.

The visualization can be done in any way—there is no right or wrong technique. If you feel you are not very adept at seeing mental imagery, use your intuition, and don't think you can't execute it. You will benefit as long as your focus is on the workout.

The optimum place to perform this exercise is in a place where you won't be interrupted. As you gain more experience, you'll be able to achieve the same beneficial effects in a busy setting, like the office. Your mental state should become calmer, and you should have a sense of mental release and relaxation.

Close your eyes and focus on your breath while sitting or standing. Put one hand on your upper chest and the other on your stomach to help you become aware of your breathing. When you breathe in, allow your stomach to expand forward; when you exhale, allow it to gently contract back. Get into a rhythm by breathing consistently at the same depth.

There should be little to no movement in your hand on your chest. Once more, make an effort to inhale at the same depth each time. Diaphragmatic breathing is what is meant by this.

When you're confident with this technique, try to slow down your breathing by taking a brief pause after each exhalation before you take another breath. Although at first, it could seem as though you are not breathing deeply enough, continuous practice will eventually make this slower rate feel natural.

Creating a cycle where you count to three when you take a breath in, stop, and then count to three when you exhale (or 2, or 4—whatever is comfortable for you) is frequently beneficial. This will also enable you to concentrate just on breathing without allowing any other thoughts to enter your head.

Simply dismiss any further thoughts that come to mind and return your focus to breathing and counting. For a few minutes, keep doing this. (If you do this often, the diaphragmatic muscle will start to get stronger and function appropriately, giving you a pleasant sense of relaxation all the time.)

Now turn your focus to your feet. Feel your feet as deeply as you can. Test your ability to feel each toe. Imagine roots slowly spreading out through the soles of your feet and descending into the ground. The roots are expanding quickly and penetrating the earth's surface deeply. You feel as secure as a giant oak or redwood tree right now because you are firmly rooted to the ground.

Spend some time focusing on this sense of safety and security that is rooted in the earth. Once you have firmly established the perception or feeling that you are rooted like a tree, see a cloud of brilliant light forming far above you. Your head is struck by a lightning strike from the luminous cloud, which ignites a band of dazzling white light that slowly descends from your head down your body, over your legs, and out beyond your toes.

Feel the band of light cleaning your mind as it travels over you. Your mind is being illuminated, and any unsettling or stressful thoughts you may have been having are being cleared. Up until you experience a sensation of cleansing and release from any worried thinking, repeat this image four or five times.

Finish by seeing yourself standing next to a huge, glowing waterfall. The river is glistening and teeming with life. You can feel the water running over every part of your body as you stand beneath the waterfall, relaxing you and evoking a profound sensation of serenity within you.

Test the water's flavor. Allow it to cool you off by opening your mouth and allowing it to enter. As it reverberates off the earth all around you, hear it. Your body and mind are being washed clean of tension and concern by the water, which is life itself. You should then open your eyes.

When performing the visualization, make an effort to utilize all of your senses. Use your senses of touch, taste, and hearing to make the images in your head as real as possible. Feel the water trickle down your body and listen to the splashing noise it makes.

You will benefit more if your envisioned situations are more realistic. Many people claim that employing these straightforward images frequently has very positive and calming effects. The mind is similar to a muscle in that it must periodically let go of what it is holding onto to relax.

You can use any setting or circumstance to help you relax. This is compared to "finding your happy place." Perhaps being at the beach or in a pool makes you feel relaxed. Consider going there. Just be confident that wherever you go in your head, you can find peace and tranquility.

You are allowing your mind to relax by picturing the various scenarios. Your brain will receive a signal when you close your eyes and start this process that it is time to let go of anything it has been holding onto mentally, including anxious thoughts.

To train your mind on how to let go of stress, it is important to practice this daily. With practice, you can learn to release all stress within minutes of starting the exercise. Your daily practice should take place before going to bed, as that will enable you to sleep more soundly.

Many people perform these visualizations before going to bed in a different room from their bedroom. In this manner, individuals leave the mental stress and worrisome thoughts behind them when they enter the bedroom and shut the door. Just make sure you have the chance to fully focus on your inner visions.

It is quite useful to use visualization as a stress management technique. If this vision is done correctly, you can experience a profound sense of inner tranquility. This method can help prevent an anxiety attack from starting, but it is unlikely to be effective in stopping one. It is an effective strategy for helping you get rid of feelings of general worry.

With practice, you discover that you may go days without having worried thoughts interfere with your life. This is crucial because it dramatically lowers the amount of overall anxiety you experience. Simply said, visualization is a skill you can employ to combat anxious thoughts and feelings. Let's examine several strategies for reducing excessive stress, starting with music.

CHAPTER EIGHT

A MUSIC-BASED STRESS RELIEF

Music may do wonders for reducing stress. Everyone has distinct musical preferences. The music that helps us feel at ease should be played. Stress may not be reduced by forcing yourself to sit down and listen to music for relaxation that you dislike. The impact of music as a mood enhancer and stress reliever is enormous and multifaceted.

Sounds have a significant impact on the entire energetic system of the human body; various tones and frequencies have a particular effect on the physical body and chakra centers. The benefits of someone genuinely performing or creating music themselves should receive extra attention.

Increased deep breathing is one of the first stress-reduction improvements that happen when we hear music. The body's serotonin synthesis also accelerates.

It has been discovered that playing background music as we work, appearing unconscious of the music itself, helps to lessen workplace stress. To distract you from the exorbitant pricing, many retail locations play music while you browse.

Music was found to reduce heart rates and to induce increased body temperature - an indication of the onset of relaxation. Relaxation therapy alone was less effective than relaxation therapy combined with music.

Many specialists contend that, despite our lack of awareness of it, the rhythm or beat of the music is what has a relaxing impact on us. They make the observation that we were presumably influenced by our mother's heartbeat while we were infants in the womb. Later in life, we react to calming music, probably because it reminds us of our mother's nurturing, relaxing surroundings.

One of the most calming or nerve-wracking experiences is listening to music. It can be challenging to decide what will work for an individual; most people choose to go with what they "enjoy" rather than what might be helpful.

Many unexpected things were discovered after conducting considerable research on the effects that any particular piece of music has on the physiological response system. In reality, several of the so-called meditation and relaxation recordings led to unfavorable EEG patterns that were on par with those of heavy metal and hard rock.

The surprising part was how calming a lot of Celtic, Native American, and other music genres with loud drums or flutes were. The most important discovery was that any music played live, even at modest volume levels and even if it was a little dissonant, had a very positive effect.

As we previously stated, not one type of music is suitable for everyone. Individuals have varying tastes. You must enjoy the tunes being played. A recent rest CD I purchased from Wal-Mart has worked wonders for me. It plays lovely piano music with the sound of the ocean in the background. It is incredibly calming.

One thing to keep in mind: If you're trying to unwind, it's probably not a good idea to listen to specific ballads or songs that conjure up unpleasant memories for you. The cause is clear. You're making an effort to unwind and get rid of your worrying thoughts. The last thing you want is for a depressing tune to trigger unwanted memories.

Here are some broad recommendations for using music to reduce stress.

1 Try taking a 20-minute "sound bath" to relieve tension. Play some soothing music on your stereo, then find a comfy spot on a couch or the floor close to the speakers and lie down. You can wear headphones for a more immersive experience to help you concentrate and cut out outside distractions.

2 Listen to music with a rhythm that is slower than your heart's normal rate of 72 beats per minute. Most people have found that repetitive or cyclical music is useful.

3 Permit the music to wash over you while it plays, washing away your day's stress. Concentrate on your breathing and allow it to slow down, deepen, and become regular. Focus on the space between the notes in the music to avoid overanalyzing it and to further your state of calm.

4 Instead of listening to soft, relaxing music after a long day at work, choose quicker music to get you going. AVOID SILENCE and DANCE! Whether or if you can dance well is unimportant. Simply follow the music and do what feels right. The sense of release will astound you!

5 When things get tough, turn to familiar music, like an old favorite or a childhood favorite. Often, familiarity fosters serenity.

6 Take strolls while listening to your favorite music on the walkman. Breathe in and out in time with the music. Give up to the music's pull. With the help of music, images, and movement (a brisk walk), this is a fantastic way to reduce stress.

7 You can lessen tension by listening to natural noises like ocean waves or the stillness of a dense forest. If you're close to a peaceful area of forests or the sea, consider going for a 15 to 20-minute walk. If not, numerous music stores sell recordings of these sounds. I've found this to be quite peaceful, and you should too!

Self-hypnosis is a fantastic relaxation technique that I have discovered to help me deal with my anxiety issues.

CHAPTER NINE

SELF-HYPNOSIS FOR STRESS

I remember feeling very stressed and anxious a few weeks back. Everything that could go wrong, it seemed, did. I had the impression that I was losing control.

I stumbled into a website offering a downloaded mp3 hypnotic relaxation session when I was writing a book on yoga and meditation at the time. It was the best $20 I've ever spent, and it only cost me about $20! These downloaded sessions are available for a modest cost in many locations on the internet. Self-hypnosis is a technique that you can learn on your own as well.

Finding a calm environment where you may unwind completely and hear your inner voice is the first step. Never try to force things to happen. Relax and listen with your thoughts free. Allowing that hypnotic state to develop spontaneously is key to obtaining it.

Additionally, avoid looking out for any indications that you might be hypnotized. We can assure you that if you watch out for these warning signs, you won't be able to fully unwind and enjoy the self-hypnosis benefits.

Hypnosis can be experienced in a variety of ways. Nobody's experience will be the same for everyone. But there is one thing that everyone agrees on: being hypnotized is always enjoyable! In hypnosis, there are no "bad trips." Keep in mind that self-hypnosis is a skill that you can develop, and as you do, it gets stronger and stronger.

Setting up a practice routine is an excellent idea. Depending on how busy you are and how much time you have available, allow yourself anywhere from 10 to 30 minutes. If you can, practice at the most enjoyable part of your day and when you are least likely to be interrupted by others.

The majority of people find it most effective to practice lying down in a relaxed setting with the fewest distractions possible. You might try to hide the noise with another source of sound if it bothers you while you are practicing.

If you like, play stereo music or white noise in the background. Try switching the stations on your radio receiver if, like the majority of people, you don't have a white noise maker. When you do that, you get static that sounds like white noise.

However, this requires a non-noise-canceling FM receiver that is older or less expensive. AM tuners can be used for this occasionally. This shouldn't be too loud to be distracting; it should just be in the background.

Relaxation, deepening, application of suggestions, and termination make up the four main parts of hypnotic induction.

1. Relaxation

Your initial task during the hypnotic induction is to calm your body's natural urges and relax. However, resist the urge to push your mind to unwind in any way! Physical relaxation will lead to mental relaxation.

Really deep relaxation is a skill that most people either lack or never learned how to do. However, some people can accomplish it fairly quickly. They simply let go of their stresses, allowing every muscle in their body to relax and become limp. If you fit this description, start your self-hypnosis session by relaxing completely. Give it some time. You should take your time with this.

Your self-hypnosis induction's relaxation phase can take anywhere from 30 minutes to just a few seconds to complete. It is a crucial component of the induction and shouldn't be overlooked. As your proficiency grows, you will be able to distinguish extremely relaxed states and enter them in a shockingly short period. However, as a beginner, go slowly. The time will be well spent.

The Jacobson Progressive Relaxation technique is a very well-liked deep relaxation technique. This entails contracting all of your body's major muscle groups (foot and lower leg on each side, upper leg and hip, abdomen, etc.). After a brief period of tension, release the muscle group.

2. Deepening Techniques

Your self-hypnosis induction's relaxation phase can take anywhere from 30 minutes to just a few seconds to complete. It is a crucial component of the induction and shouldn't be overlooked. As your proficiency grows, you will be able to distinguish extremely relaxed states and enter them in a shockingly short period. However, as a beginner, go slowly. The time will be well spent.

The Jacobson Progressive Relaxation technique is a very well-liked deep relaxation technique. This entails contracting all of your body's major muscle groups (foot and lower leg on each side, upper leg and hip, abdomen, etc.). After a brief period of tension, release the muscle group.

If you don't remove the thought of watching for hypnosis out of your head, it will undoubtedly get in the way. In this way, entering a hypnotic trance is analogous to falling asleep. You are considerably less likely to fall asleep if you strive to catch yourself doing it—if you try to be conscious of the precise second when you do fall asleep. You can't sleep while "watching."

Similarly, you won't be able to recognize when you enter a hypnotic state (although you won't be able to because you won't have lost consciousness). After a few weeks or months of consistent practice, you'll be much more familiar with yourself and how it feels to be hypnotized.

Does everyone require weeks or even months to reach a nice trance state? Not. Some people encounter it for the first time in an extraordinary way. Others may practice for a few days without recognizing anything, and then all of a sudden have one of those fantastic induction periods during which they suddenly realize something extraordinarily positive occurred. However, if you're not one of them, don't stress about it. You'll succeed if you just keep working at it.

The count-down approach is one of the most widely used deepening techniques. This one is also popular in Hollywood. That explains why it appears in so many films. Along with the watch that swings.

Simply begin counting down from, say, 20, to employ the count-down approach (or 100, or whatever). After some practice, change the countdown number to whatever seems comfortable to you. Imagine that with each count, you are descending more. As you count, more images and ideas will likely enter your head. That makes sense. Continue counting while you kindly sweep them aside.

You should count down at a natural pace that is neither too fast nor too sluggish. For the majority of people, this entails counting roughly every two or three seconds. Work at a pace that is easy and comfortable for you. Some individuals like to relate the count to breathing. Their breathing slows down as they float deeper, which causes their counting to slow down as well.

Just mentally work your way down the count; don't count aloud. You want to limit your physical activity and movement as much as possible.

3. Application of Suggestions in Self-Hypnosis

When your process of deepening is complete, you are prepared to put the advice into practice. Your suggestibility has increased as a result of the relaxing and deepening techniques. In other words, you have at least slightly allowed your suggestions to enter your subconscious mind. This works as a result of the unique and peculiar qualities of your subconscious mind.

The most frequent and simple approach to putting advice into practice is to have it figured out beforehand, correctly phrased, and memorized. They should be quite brief, and since you wrote them, it shouldn't be too difficult to recall them. You can just mentally work your way through them at this point if you have them prepared and in mind.

It's also acceptable to have a monologue or dialogue. To make the least amount of effort, you simply think (or "speak") to yourself about what you want to do, be, or become.

Avoid using "you." Use the first person personal pronoun "I" since you are thinking to yourself. Some advice can be briefly expressed in a little more formal manner, such as, "I am eating less and getting leaner every day."

In general, elaborate recommendations are longer and more impromptu: "Every day, I place less importance on food and fill my time with activities that are more worthwhile and significant. Desserts and other fatty foods are getting easier and easier to avoid." so forth.

In general, image suggestion is the most successful type of suggestion. Typically, image ideas don't use any text at all. This might be compared to picturing yourself in a peaceful, calm condition amid a hectic circumstance. Take a mental picture of yourself.

Even while people occasionally notice an instant impact from their suggestions, it usually takes some time for them to take effect. So try not to rush things. On the other hand, you should revise your recommendations if you haven't started to see any outcomes after, say, a couple of weeks.

4. Termination

You have completed your induction when you have finished implementing the advice, at which point you can end the session. You could simply open your eyes, stand up, and carry on with your day, but it is not recommended.

The conclusion of every session should be declared in writing. By doing this, you establish a distinct separation between your normal conscious awareness and the hypnotic state. Additionally, a distinct end to your self-hypnosis practice session stops it from morphing into a snooze. Take a snooze if you feel like it. However, avoid doing so in a way that links practicing self-hypnosis with sleeping.

It's acceptable to practice before going to sleep if you don't care if you stay asleep. Draw the boundary for the end of your self-hypnosis session nonetheless. Think to yourself that you will be fully awake and attentive when you count up to, say, three to end the session.

"One, I'm starting to emerge from it and am heading toward waking up. Two, I'm starting to wake up and am becoming more awake. Third, I'm fully awake." equivalent to that

When self-hypnosis is used frequently, it can be quite effective. You'd be astonished at the degree of relaxation you can get. One of the best things I've ever done for myself, I should add.

We should now discuss general stress management strategies. This chapter may be lengthy, but it is quite beneficial.

CHAPTER TEN

MANAGEMENT OF STRESS

Stress is a part of life, as we have previously stated. Nothing can be done to avoid it. Some stress is beneficial. You might not believe it, but occasionally stress can inspire us to take actions that we might not typically take when we're calm. When we are under stress, we can muster the courage to act when we otherwise might hesitate.

To successfully manage stress and allow it to improve our lives rather than control them, we need to be resilient. How can one become tough and resilient? By understanding how to manage your stress and turn it into an asset rather than a liability.

Recognizing stress signs can be helpful since it motivates us to act, and the sooner the better. The death of a loved one, the birth of a child, a job promotion, or the beginning of a new relationship is some of the more frequent occurrences that cause those emotions. However, it's not always simple to determine why you feel stressed in each case. As we restructure our life, we feel stress. When you experience these signs of stress, your body is pleading with you to assist it.

In this chapter, we're going to provide a lot of recommendations for you. We're ready to wager that some of them will, even though not all of them will work for you.

To handle stress, there are three main strategies. The first is an approach that focuses on action. With this approach, the issues that lead to stress are identified, and the appropriate adjustments are made for a life free of stress.

The following strategy is emotionally focused, and in it, the person manages stress by providing the situation that stressed them a new perspective. The stressful circumstance is viewed in a humorous or alternative light.

I particularly support this method of stress reduction. If you don't laugh at a scenario, you might start sobbing hysterically sometimes. That is not a remedy. So train your eyes to perceive laughter rather than gloom.

The third strategy is acceptance-focused. This strategy focuses on handling tension that was brought on by a former issue.

The first stress-reduction advice is to identify the underlying causes of your stress. Nobody knows your issue better than you do. Spending a few minutes to identify your genuine emotions can completely alter the scenario.

Determine the cause of the tension during this process. Share it with a loved one nearby if they are present. Take a deep breath and count to ten if you are feeling overly overwhelmed and on the verge of collapsing. This revitalizes the entire body by pumping more oxygen into it.

When under extreme stress, take a moment to meditate and step outside of the immediate environment. From your current position, get up and start walking. Attempt to stretch. You'll soon notice that the stress has reduced.

This is because you are currently calm, which is the best stress reliever. Another technique for managing stress is to smile. Simply get up and grin at your coworker in the opposite corner if you're at work. Your mood will alter, you'll notice. Pick up some basic yoga or meditation skills.

You can also come up with your stress-reduction strategies. The fundamental concept is to pinpoint the source of stress, take a break from it for a while, and then address it. Another method of reducing stress is to take a quick stroll while admiring natural objects. Simple stress-reduction tactics include drinking a glass of water and playing quick games. The aim is to shift your attention away from the issue so that when you return to it, it won't seem as overwhelming as it did before.

Five quick actions you can take to reduce stress are listed below:

1. Don't just stand still. Move! Many psychologists believe that motion elicits emotion. You could have noticed that it's simpler to get depressed when you're not doing anything. You droop in a chair, lowering your heart rate, decreasing the amount of oxygen getting to your brain, and preventing air from getting to your lungs.

Regardless of how you are feeling right now, I dare you to get up and move quickly. Perhaps you should enter an unoccupied room and hop around a little bit. Although it may seem absurd, the outcomes speak for themselves. Right away, give it a try. It works enchantment.

A fantastic way to reduce stress is to exercise. A panic episode during aerobic activity may scare those with anxiety disorders. After all, as you exercise, your breathing gets heavier, your heart rate increases, and you start sweating.

It's not an attack, so don't freak out! While you are working out, keep telling yourself this. Recognize that there is a significant distinction between what happens when you work out and the physical side of it.

2. Take a moment to breathe in the blooms. How do you take a whiff of roses? Consider investing to fund the vacation you've always wanted to take. Visit an exotic location-rich nation to spark your imagination and inspire your creativity. You must step away from your routine and travel a little.

3. Assist others in solving their challenges. When you immerse yourself in helping others, it is immensely soothing. You'd be shocked at how many people have issues that are more serious than yours. There are various ways in which you can help others. Don't let stress and depression cause you to cuddle up in bed.

Get outside and assist someone. But take care. Avoid getting sucked into other people's issues to ignore your own.

Friends and family call me frequently when they need to vent or seek advice. Don't call the "crazy" individual for advice, I jokingly advise.

However, there are instances when I find myself thinking about the people that call me and I become preoccupied with their problems. I realize that I need to take a break and reevaluate my priorities because this only adds to my already high level of stress.

Now I can tell them to call back later because I'm just not able to handle it right now. They occasionally become agitated, but more often than not, they comprehend. I've learned, though, not to let their responses get to me. It should matter now even if it won't matter in a week.

4. Have a little fun. You've probably already heard that laughter is a healthy internal remedy. It relaxes the muscles and releases tension. Blood starts to flow to the heart and brain as a result. More significantly, laughing causes the production of a substance that relieves pain in the body.

Researchers learn new advantages of laughter every day. Can you occasionally benefit from a good dose of belly-shaking laughter? You can, of course. What are you holding out for? Rent some amusing movies or visit a comedy club.

5. Exhaust your knees. If I could give you one lasting solution when things get rough, it would be prayer. Depending on their religion, many individuals may refer to it as meditation. What you call it doesn't matter to me as long as you have somewhere to flee to.

You now have a few options for immediate stress relief. Need more? No issue!

CHAPTER ELEVEN

ADDITIONAL STRESS MANAGEMENT

Make anxiety your friend.

Make stress your buddy and acknowledge its benefits! The body's natural "fight or flight" response will cause that energy to burst to improve your performance when it matters most. A top athlete who was completely at ease before a major competition has yet to be seen. When it matters most, use stress to your advantage and push yourself a little bit harder.

Stress spreads easily

This means that negative people can cause a lot of stress. Stress is bred by negativity, and some people only know how to whine. Now, there are two ways to approach this. They hope that you can help them get back "up" because they first perceive you as a pleasant, happy person. If not, they are simply a pessimistic individual who is unable to feel better about themselves unless those around them share their viewpoints.

Avoid getting sucked into their behavior of downing. Limit your contact with these folks after realizing that they deal with stress on their own. You might try to play stress doctor and teach them better stress management techniques but tread carefully as this could increase your stress levels more.

Model effective stress management techniques

Who remains composed when everyone else is losing their cool? What exactly are they changing? What attitude do they have? What dialect do they speak? Are they skilled and knowledgeable?

Determine it from a distance or have a conversation with them. Study the most effective stress reducers and do as they say.

Take deep breaths.

By inhaling deeply, you can deceive your body into relaxing. Take a slow seven-count inhalation and an eleven-count exhalation. Repeat the 7-11 breathing exercise until your heart rate decreases, your sweat-covered hands stop, and you begin to feel more normal.

Put an end to anxious thoughts

You could get yourself all by yourself into a stress knot. "If this occurs, that may occur, and then we're all in deep water!" Why expend all that energy worrying needlessly when the majority of these things never happen?

Give stressful thoughts the red light and put a stop to them. It could go wrong, but how likely is that to happen and what can you do to prevent it?

Know your triggers and stress hotspots.

Delivering challenging comments, dealing with clients, presenting presentations, meeting deadlines, etc. The mere act of penning them down has my heart racing.

Make a list of your stress hot spots or trigger points. Be precise. Do speeches to particular audiences seem to rile you up more than others? Do certain projects stress people out more than others? Have you consumed too much coffee?

Knowing what makes you stressed out is useful information since you can take steps to reduce your stress. Do you need to pick up any new abilities? Are further resources required? Should you switch to decaffeinated coffee instead?

Eat, drink, rest, and have fun!

Our body and mind suffer greatly when we are sleep deprived, eat poorly, or do not exercise. Kind of obvious, but important to highlight because it's frequently overlooked as a stress-reduction method. Don't burn the candle at both ends; instead, pay attention to your mother!

Stay away from artificial stress relief methods. This means that you shouldn't instinctively pour a drink of wine or smoke a cigarette when you feel yourself starting to become agitated. Substances like alcohol, cigarettes, caffeine, and narcotics can exacerbate the issue. Practicing the relaxing methods we've given you instead would be a better option. You can then have that glass of wine if you'd like once you're at ease.

Step outside and take in the scenery. A little sunshine and exercise can have a remarkable impact on your stress level and improve your view of life as a whole. Everyone in your family and/or circle of friends will benefit from your improved attitude, and problems that first seemed overwhelming will fade into insignificance, leaving you wondering what the problem was.

You won't just feel less stressed; you'll also be better for it—healthier, happier, and more energized—and prepared to take on any challenges that come your way.

Permit yourself to act like a child once more. What did you like to do as a kid? Be imaginative; draw, paint, etc. Play around dance, play-dough, or reading. Play some music and express yourself without worrying about conforming to society's expectations of who you "should" be. Just unwind and have fun. We all have a little child inside of us, and it's a good idea to occasionally let that child out to play.

If I may say so, this advice is great and extremely healing. I can talk from experience. Nothing makes me happier than purchasing a brand-new box of 64 Crayons—the kind with the sharpener inside the box—and drawing endlessly in a coloring book. When I use this stress reliever, my grandson adores it!

Avoid setting yourself up for failure by doing so. By giving ourselves unattainable goals, many of us unwittingly set ourselves up for failure. Realize that you cannot drop 40 pounds in just one or two months, for instance, if you are dieting.

Or perhaps your goal is to get a specific job position; whatever your objective, give yourself enough time to accomplish it and be aware that failures occasionally happen.

You will feel even better about yourself if you accomplish your objective without encountering any obstacles, but don't count on it. In actuality, don't have any expectations; reality frequently differs greatly from expectations.

1. Acquire the ability to occasionally say "no." Many of us frequently believe that we must always answer positively to requests for assistance and feel that we must always say "yes" to everyone. But keep in mind that you cannot please everyone. Before you can fully offer others what they need while keeping yourself happy, you must first take care of your own needs.

2. You are not required to comply with all requests from your family, friends, and others. Yes, you should assist others, but only after you have taken the necessary steps to look after yourself.

3. Give yourself the attention you deserve. Once your needs are addressed, you'll find that you have more time for others. And if you don't feel that you have to continually put other people's needs ahead of your own, you might enjoy helping others more.

We're still not done! There are countless effective methods for overcoming stress and anxiety. You have a right to learn everything you can. After all, isn't it the main reason you're reading this book? Here are some other stress relievers.

CHAPTER TWELVE

WHO DID YOU RING? STRESS RELIEVERS!

1. I've personally utilized this idea a lot and appreciate it! Yell! Yes, scream as loudly as you can, at the top of your lungs. Even while you might not be able to accomplish this at home, it works perfectly when you're driving with the windows down. yelled guttural from the bottom of my soul. It liberates you!

2. Sing. As we mentioned in the last chapter, listening to music can be a very effective way to relieve tension. Imagine how much better you'll feel if you sing "Copacabana" loud and proud! Who gives a damn if you can't sing? You're pursuing this for yourself!

3. Start a new activity, such as knitting or crocheting. Don't stress about doing it well. The method itself is advantageous. For many people, remaining motionless while executing repetitive movements is calming and stabilizing. It might be time for you to gather your thoughts.

4. Start a garden, Apartment residents can also accomplish this. Potted plants can be found inside, outside, or in a small area of your yard. It takes a little effort to set up.

5. It's rewarding to take care of plants, fruits, veggies, and flowers and watch them grow, bloom, or provide food. The best approach to manage tension and concern, according to ardent gardeners, is to work in the garden. The improvement of the environment's beauty and tranquility is a bonus.

6. Have fun with a cat or dog. According to experts, pet owners live longer and have fewer signs of stress than non-pet owners. Playing with your pet is healthy for both you and the animal! It's a sort of social connection where you're not under any obligation to please anyone!

7. Take a look at the moon and the stars. Observing the night sky while lying on a blanket with your hands behind your head may be

incredibly humbling. It's not just humble; it's also incredibly lovely and soothing.

My grandson and I recently spread a blanket out in the yard to watch the moon set behind the clouds and to look at the stars. Seeing the sky through his eyes made it even more intriguing for me. He is only three years old, so it is a great experience for him.

We talked about astronauts who get to view the stars up close and how the universe is vast while we are still so small, and I felt all my anxieties wash away. The vastness of the sky makes you realize how insignificant our troubles are in comparison. I also find immense comfort in the fact that there is always one bright star above my house

After leaving the funeral for my best friend's mother, we got out of the car and I paused to look at the stars with my friend's five-year-old. "That's my grandma," she replied, pointing to a certain star. She is now our protector angel. I can always count on Cheryl to get me through anything when I see that star.

8. Indulge in some comfort food. But take care, as overeating could end up being your main source of stress. Enjoy it in moderation to boost your mood.

I adore mac and cheese, mashed potatoes, and gravy. My go-to comfort foods are those. But I watch that I don't go overboard. I only give myself enough to elicit that relaxing sensation.

9. Swing. Remember how it felt to be swaying back and forth within that tiny piece of leather on the playground with the wind ruffling your hair? Try it! If your yard doesn't have a swing, visit a playground and keep in mind to pump your legs to see how high you can go. It liberates you!

10. Have a bubble bath with candles. Even you guys out there could use a warm bath filled with the calming glow of candles. When you pull the plug, lay back, enjoy the warm water and bubbles, and let all of your worries drain away.

Phew! There you have it—27 techniques to unwind and reduce stress. You are also free to devise your solutions! Finding a coping mechanism that works for you when you're overwhelmed and doing it consistently is the key. Your general health will improve.

CHAPTER THIRTEEN

SIMPLY SAY "NO"

The ability to say "No" when necessary is a big issue for those who are unduly stressed. Perhaps your mother asks you to take Grandma to the grocery, but you're working on a significant assignment at work right now. When you've already made plans with yourself to get a haircut, perhaps your best friend asks if you'd mind watching her children.

You are not required to accept everyone's invitations. In reality, there are numerous occasions when you should decline their invitations. You are a people pleaser if you frequently find yourself saying "yes" to requests that you don't want to make. Although this isn't a bad trait in general, it can be extremely stressful.

People-pleasers put the needs of others ahead of their own. Others spend a lot of time serving the needs of others and worry constantly about what they desire, think, or need. They rarely take care of their own needs and feel bad when they do. Being a people-pleaser is challenging.

People-pleasers are reluctant to express their true opinions or request what they need because they fear offending others. However, they frequently interact with people who are completely uninterested in their needs. People-pleasers frequently feel compelled to cheer up insensitive or sad others, even at their own expense.

It is exhausting to constantly try to please others, and many people pleasers frequently experience feelings of anxiety, worry, unhappiness, and fatigue. Even though they give so much to others and may not understand why they receive nothing in return, they frequently refuse to ask for what they require.

This is the trap I got caught in. Every time I offered to help someone else, I discovered that when I needed those same folks to assist ME, they were mysteriously preoccupied.

A people-pleaser might think that if they ask for assistance and the other person agrees, they are only doing it out of obligation and not out of genuine desire. It is believed that if they truly intended to assist, they would have done it without my request.

This style of thinking develops because people-pleasers themselves feel obligated to lend a hand and don't always act out of pure motivation. Unfortunately, people-pleasers have been taught that their value is based on what they do for other people.

Being a people pleaser is painful—trust me, I know! People-pleasers frequently take things personally, are very sensitive to other people's feelings, and rarely put their own needs first.

They are frequently on the move, hurrying to complete tasks because when they do take some time for themselves, they feel egotistical, indulgent, and guilty. People pleasers are generally the first to be asked to do things, which makes them open to being used because they accomplish so much and are easy to get along with.

Most likely, people pleasers were raised in households where their needs and feelings were not acknowledged, respected, or given much weight. When they were young, they frequently had to meet or tend to the needs of others. Alternatively, they might have been hushed, neglected, or subjected to various forms of maltreatment, learning that their needs and feelings were unimportant.

Girls are taught in many cultures to be people-pleasers who put the needs of others before their own. There is at least some element of people-pleasing in many women. Men who related to their mothers frequently did so as well.

People pleasers tend to put more of their attention on others than on themselves. They frequently feel empty or are unsure about their feelings, thoughts, or personal goals. However, it is possible to break this tendency and improve your self-esteem.

I was able to figure out how to stop this loop. If you identify with the preceding description, you can take the same action. You're curious about how. It's simpler than you would imagine!

Practice saying no first. This word is significant! Just to hear the word come out of your mouth, repeat it as much as you can. When you are by yourself, say it out. Practice saying "No, I can't do that" or "No, I don't want to go there," among other NO-containing sentences. Try it out for easy scenarios first, and work your way up to more challenging ones.

You shouldn't constantly say "yes." Before responding to someone's request, try pausing or taking a deep breath. The phrase "I need to think about it first, I'll get back to you" or "Let me check my schedule and call you back" are possible responses to requests. Use any term that gives you time before automatically answering "YES" and that you feel comfortable using.

Take brief pauses, despite your guilt. Although you won't constantly feel guilty, you probably will at first. Keep in mind that the annoyance you might have to endure from others is well worth maintaining your mental wellness. You are what's crucial. Everyone around you will be healthy if you are!

Find out what makes you happy. For instance, you might enjoy listening to music, visiting parks, viewing videos, or reading periodicals. Give yourself the go-ahead to do such things, then take pleasure in them.

Request assistance from someone. Although I realize it's challenging, you can accomplish it! Why shouldn't YOU ask THEM if everyone else is asking YOU for favors? Just be understanding if they reject you. Simply because you've always said "yes," doesn't mean they have to reciprocate.

Become aware of your thoughts and feelings. These things are significant to be aware of since they define who you are. Then, try expressing your thoughts and feelings more frequently. Just be mindful to maintain some civility when necessary.

Many people-pleasers think that if they stop doing things for other people, no one would like them. You're being exploited by someone if they cease like you because you refuse to do what they want, and you probably don't want them as a friend anyhow.

People will like you not just for what you do, but also for who you are. You have the right to put yourself first, to refuse requests from others, and to take care of yourself without feeling guilty. One little step at a time, you can make a change.

The majority of people, I believe, would agree wholeheartedly with what I have to say next. McDonald's was right when they said, "You Deserve A Break Today!"

CHAPTER FOURTEEN

QUIT AND RELAX

We frequently recognize deep down that we need a break. That break could be a long vacation or a quick weekend trip. In either case, escaping the daily grind may be incredibly liberating and a significant means of reducing stress and anxiety.

Sadly, a lot of individuals believe they can't take the time to travel. This is a harmful mentality. Get outside and leave!

How frequently have you kept working despite knowing that you weren't giving the job your all? How many times have you read or written the same phrase over while your mind was off thinking about something else? How many times have you wanted to take a break from your family or children but were afraid of the repercussions? Time for a break, please!

Why don't we permit ourselves to take a "time out"? It's possible that we believe we don't deserve it or that there is simply too much to do. There are numerous valid motivations to finish work and duties, but occasionally we may also have "hidden agendas" for why we cannot take a vacation. Why?

Maybe it's ego. Some individuals only take pleasure in bragging about "how late they had to work to accomplish a project" or "how much effort they committed to do the job so swiftly." This kind of person frequently seeks to impress people with their work to boost their ego.

You could believe that you simply cannot take the time off. I have to finish this; I can't quit now. This may sound familiar to you. "Because the work must be completed, I am unable to stop. WHY? For me to immediately go on to the next task, and the next, and the next, etc." This individual will discover that there is always work to be done, which prevents them from taking breaks frequently.

Perhaps you merely have the urge to be needed. A mother running a home, raising children, and doing other tasks could feel as though her home would fall apart if she took a weekend off. She can maintain telling herself that her contribution is essential and that the family would split apart if she takes a break by refusing to do so. This might be the case, but that doesn't make it a good enough excuse to keep her from taking a nap.

Get that idea out of your head! By spending a little time for yourself, you can reap some incredible rewards. Resting your mind and/or body can help you refocus your attention, improve your reasoning, and boost your motivation. Additionally, taking a break can aid in the recuperation of tired muscles, ease stress, and encourage the realization that life is about more than just work.

Many athletes will tell you that rest is an essential component of their training regimen. After a workout, muscles require some time to recover. Keep in mind that your brain functions similarly to muscles. To function at its optimum, it requires time to rest and recover. You'll be able to focus better and give tasks you once found challenging your complete attention if you give your brain some downtime. Believe me, they will be simpler!

You've therefore determined that a break is necessary. Bravo to you! From a 10-minute meditation session to a trip around the world and everything in between, a break may be anything. I believe a break should involve something that diverts attention from the daily boredom of life

Therefore, depending on how much time you have available for relaxation, you might like to read, watch a movie, cook, play with the kids, ride a motorcycle or drive, exercise or engage in sports, go on a trip, or just sleep!

Above all, permit yourself to take this break when you need it, and don't feel bad about it. Take advantage of this time off because you will benefit so much from it.

Contrary to what your mind may be telling you, everyone will live even without you! Life will go on without you! Allow yourself to let go of everything and focus on YOU once instead of everyone else!

Don't be a martyr or think less of yourself if you're feeling exhausted, unmotivated, or simply in need of a break. You might discover that, in the long run, giving yourself a break will help you become more effective in every aspect of your life. Additionally, you will receive the much-needed and merited "batteries" recharging!

One of the locations that might be the most stressful is the workplace. When you're around your coworkers, you could believe that none of these strategies can be of any use to you. You are utterly mistaken.

CHAPTER FIFTEEN

RELAXING AT WORK

You can take a break from work at other times as well, not just during coffee breaks. My experience has shown me that taking coffee (or smoking) breaks during the workday might make you feel more stressed.

While some of the advice we've given you in this book can be put into effect at the office, regrettably, some cannot. Here is a tried-and-true technique to aid with your workplace relaxation.

Find a place to sit first, of course. Put your feet level on the floor, sit up straight, and place your hands lightly on your thighs with your back on the back of the chair.

Close your eyes if you can. Even while you can perform the exercise without closing your eyes, doing so will make you feel a little more relaxed. Avoid closing your eyes tightly. Your eyelids should naturally close.

Slowly inhale through your nose while counting to five. For five counts, hold your breath. Exhale slowly while counting to five. Repeat.

A set of muscles must be tensed and held for a count of 5, then released for a count of 5, to complete this exercise.

Do your best to avoid being harmed when you contract each group of muscles. Be as calm as you can when you relinquish the hold.

Tension your feet first. To do this, lift your feet off the ground and point your toes in the direction of your body while keeping your heels on the ground. Hold for a slow five counts. Let go of the grip. Allow your feet to softly recline. Feel the calmness. Consider how it differs from when you clenched your muscles. Unwind for five counts.

Next, contract your thigh muscles as tightly as possible. Hold for five counts. Calm your body and count to five.

Your abs should be tight, so keep that position for five counts. For five counts, let your muscles relax. Make sure you are still sitting up properly.

Squeeze your hands into fists as tightly as you can to tense your arm and hand muscles. Hold for five counts. For a count of five, thoroughly relax your muscles.

Pushing your shoulders back and attempting to touch your shoulder blades together can help you to tighten your upper back. Hold for five counts. Unwind for five counts.

Raise your shoulders toward your ears in a shrugging motion, then hold for five counts. Unwind for five counts.

First, gently tilt your head back while holding for five seconds to tighten your neck. unwind for five. After then, gently tilt your head forward for five seconds. Unwind for five counts.

Face muscles should be contracted. first, widen your mouth for five seconds. unwind for five. Then, raise your eyebrows and hold them there for 5 seconds. unwind for five. Finally, close your eyes firmly and hold for five seconds. 5 minutes of calm (with your eyes slightly closed).

With breathing, the workout is completed. Slowly inhale through your nose while counting to five. For five counts, hold your breath. Exhale slowly while counting to five. 4) Repetition. That's all, then!

Anytime you need to unwind, whether you're in a car, on a plane, or wherever else you could be sitting, do this practice. This practice shouldn't be done while driving because it might be quite calming.

If you do this exercise consistently over time, you will learn to notice tightness in your body. You won't have to do the entire exercise; you can relax your muscles whenever you like. For long-term outcomes, exercise at least twice each day.

By using more muscle groups, you can create a relaxation exercise that lasts longer. Identify your stress points and alternately tense them and release them.

By picturing a serene environment after the exercise, you can maximize the relaxation advantages. Spend at least five minutes picturing in great detail a setting where you feel at ease. Do you recall the pleasant place? Visit it and have fun!

CONCLUSION

We hope you grasp and comprehend that there is NO WAY to entirely eradicate stress from your life if you take nothing else away from reading this book. What you can do is figure out how to use that tension to your advantage.

It's not as difficult to manage stress as it may appear. But we cannot stress this following point enough. Consult your physician, a spiritual guide, or a local mental health organization if you feel that your life is too stressful. They could advise you to consult a psychiatrist, psychologist, social worker, or another skilled counselor because responses to stress can play a role in depression, anxiety, and other illnesses.

We don't want to come across as experts in medicine. All we're trying to do is provide you with some tools you can use to deal with the things that overwhelm you and make us feel out of control in your life.

To reduce some of your stress, you might also want to look into time management software. You don't want to experience anxiety if you feel like you don't have enough time to complete the tasks at hand. This increases stress.

Simple, inexpensive strategies to effectively reduce stress include stress management techniques. They can be used at any time and anywhere. Well, nearly!

Do not hesitate to seek assistance if you think you need it. You might not always be right. Your tension may be coming from absolutely nothing. But its origins could be physical. It can be a simple problem for someone else to resolve. Recognizing your limitations can significantly reduce stress.

The stress of everyday living is common. Stress is beneficial in moderation since it can spur motivation and increase output. But excessive stress or a strong stress reaction might be dangerous.

It can make you more susceptible to both general ill health and particular physical or mental conditions like infection, heart disease, or depression. Stress that is constant and severe can cause anxiety as well as undesirable habits like overeating and drug or alcohol abuse.

The things that relieve stress vary from person to person, just as the causes of stress do. However, most people find it helpful to make some lifestyle adjustments and to find pleasurable, healthy methods to deal with stress. I hope I've provided you with some excellent strategies for coping with the stress we all experience!

Above all, keep in mind that you are not fighting this struggle by yourself. There are countless numbers of people who feel absolutely out of control and overwhelmed. We wanted to send you this book for that reason. So that you might discover inner peace and understand why everyone is on this great blue marble.

Also, you are! Live life to the fullest and take it all in. And when you experience stress or a panic attack, remember to breathe through it and to relax since a great many other people can relate to how you're feeling.

"Don't Worry, Be Happy" is Bobby McFerrin's motto, which I find to be the best overall.

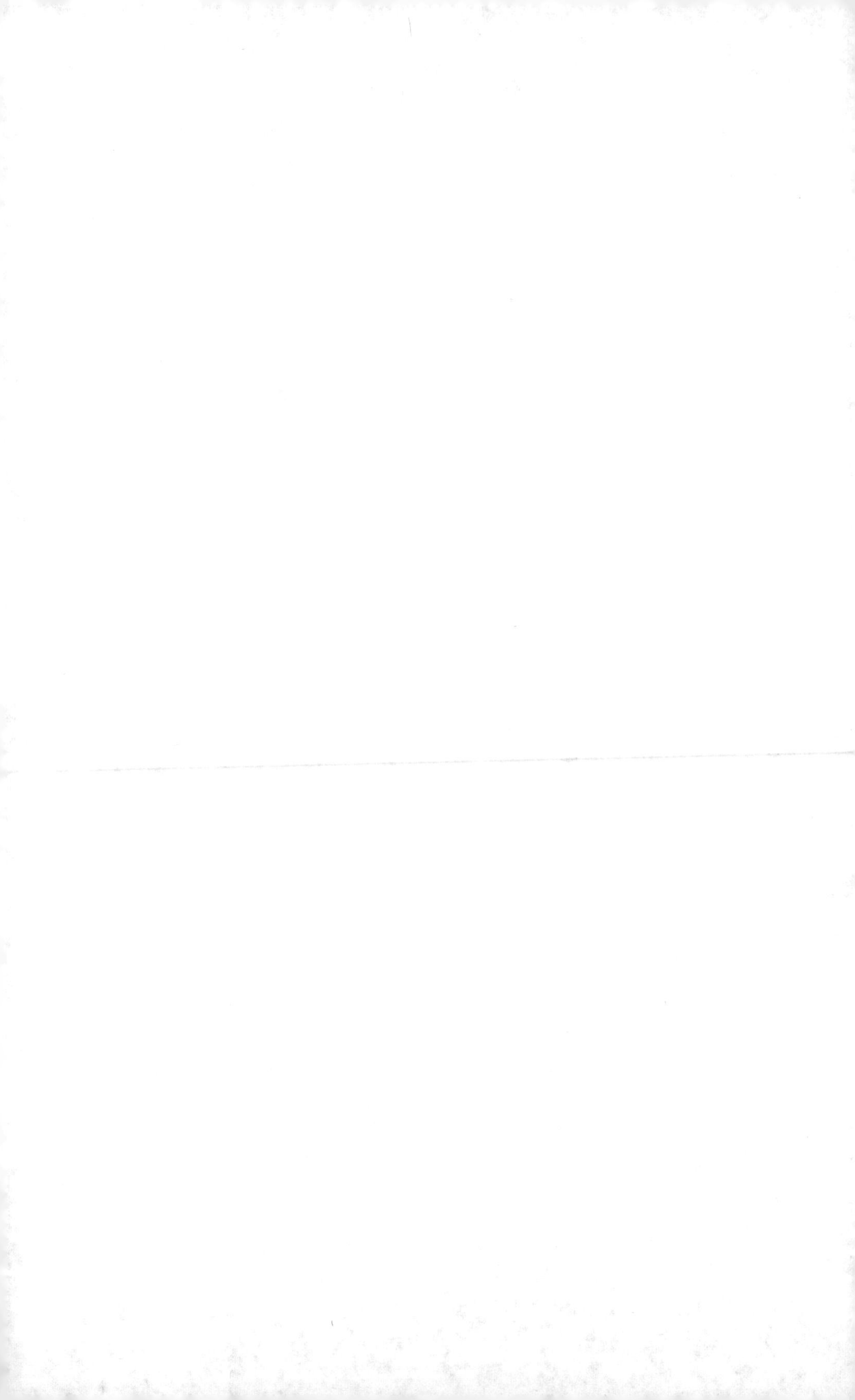

www.ingramcontent.com/pod-product-compliance
Lightning Source LLC
Chambersburg PA
CBHW051702250726
48653CB00007B/2810